Intermittent Fasting Diet Plan

How to Master the Act of Fasting for a Better Body

By J. Steele

RWG Publishing

PO Box 596

Litchfield, IL 62056

https://rwgpublishing.com/

Published in the United States of America

Contents

Introduction

Intermittent fasting has been gaining a positive reputation over the years and for a good reason. Not only does science show that this way of eating can bring great health benefits, but hundreds of people I have guided with my teachings have approved of this method. More energy, faster fat burning and a younger appearance are just some of the benefits of fasting. In this book, I'll show you how intermittent fasting works, how you can reap the benefits as well as warn you about some potential drawbacks.

If you want a quick way to lose weight, then this diet plan is the way to go. Intermittent fasting will make you shed unwanted body fat in no time as well as reap some unbelievable health benefits! I have carefully outlined all types of intermittent fasting schedules that you can easily follow in these chapters. This book will be your best companion on your journey to a better and slimmer body. Make sure to take things slow with one step at a time and I know you will reach your ideal weight goals. All is possible. Happy fasting!

Chapter 1

What is Intermittent Fasting?

Intermittent fasting is a form of alternating fasting. This type of fasting will give you extremely beneficial health effects and is effective for weight loss. Intermittent fasting involves eating only for a few hours a day on a regular basis (every day or several times a week) and refrain from eating for the rest of the day. There are several variations to this diet plan ranging from 16 hours of fasting to several days of fasting (which is quite extreme). Intermittent fasting can help you lose weight faster and has a lot of health benefits, but beware! It's not for everyone!

What is Intermittent Fasting?

Intermittent fasting gives you a healthy dose of stress that puts your body back into *survival mode*. Think of this scenario as if you were living during prehistoric times. Your body may think there is an energy shortage and needs to be fit and ready for the hunt which often takes a lot of time and energy. This energy burns up your fat supply (which is why you lose weight immediately during fasting!). Your body will also make an effort to resolve inflammation quickly as it did for those prehistoric hunters. Fasting every other day means that you eat very little one day (less than 25% of your energy requirement) alternated with a day on which you can eat everything. Periodic fasting means that you fast from food 1 to 2 days a week. You can also fast for a certain number of hours a day. A well-known example of this is called *Ramadan fasting*. The intermittent fasting plan is a diet that allows for quick weight loss, more energy and other positive health benefits.

Intermittent fasting or interval fasting emphasizes not on what you eat but *when* you eat. One example: you can eat between 12:00PM and 8:00PM and refrain from eating the rest of the day. With this method, you fast from food for 16 hours in a row. With this fasting method, you will experience several positive effects including weight loss, increased resistance and a natural energetic boost.

Intermittent fasting also amounts to eating only at certain times of the day or week, and then nothing at all at other times. One example is allowing yourself to eat between 11:00AM and 7:00PM, and you fast from food until 11:00AM the following day. Later in this book, you will find an overview of the different intermittent fasting diet plans that are available. During your individual time of fasting, I recommend drinking water, coffee or tea. I also recommend that you follow a low-carb, natural and unprocessed diet when you do eat. That way you get the most out of all the benefits of intermittent fasting.

Isn't intermittent fasting a bit extreme?

You are probably used to eating 3 meals a day along with a snack here and there and now I challenge you to a completely different schedule. With some intermittent fasting diet plans, you only eat 1 meal a day which will take some getting used to, especially in the beginning. Just a warning, with the more extreme fasting diet plans, you may experience:

- An increased feeling of hunger and more of an appetite for snacks
- Irritation or feeling moody, shivering or physical weakness
- Less energy and fatigue, especially during physically intensive activities (i.e. playing sports)

Most people who fast are completely used to their new eating rhythm after two weeks. You may still experience a feeling of hunger while fasting, but the deep longing for food is not nearly as intense as the first week. The food you choose to consume has a significant influence on the degree to which you experience any discomfort during your time of fasting. The healthier you eat, the less physical or emotional discomfort you will feel as your fasting diet continues.

Intermittent fasting; healthier and easier than you may think

I am skilled at sharing all this information because last year, I was on a specific diet plan and discovered the power of intermittent fasting. I had read all kinds of scientific studies about fasting and felt confident as I started applying the fasting principles in my own life. Honestly, I don't like fasting at all, but this diet plan turned out to be much easier than I realized and I feel really good about the effects on my mind and body. Intermittent fasting means you occasionally skip one or more meals. More and more people are discovering greater weight loss and increased energy through the power of intermittent fasting. There is also scientific research that indicates that grazing for cows is fine every day but not as necessary for humans.

Processing food is hard work for your body

Your body has to process more and naturally work every time you eat. Your body is beautifully balanced and when you constantly eat several meals a day, that natural balance gets disrupted and your body must once again work out the process to regain internal balance. In fact, everything you eat is *foreign*. Your digestive system immediately starts digesting and processing food you consume and removing any useless food particles. This is quite an effort! It is always a good idea to give your body occasional rest by refraining from eating.

Chapter 2

The Science behind Fasting

Intermittent fasting is a diet plan you may hear about more often these days. The three most popular forms of intermittent fasting are: fasting every other day, fasting 2 days a week or daily eating within a fixed time period (time-restrictive eating). Not only does weight loss occur, which can lead to better health, many other benefits are also experienced. An extensive article in the New England Journal of Medicine revealed the mechanism, benefits, and application of intermittent fasting and some of these facts I will discuss in these chapters. I will touch on the benefits of intermittent fasting in later chapters but now I want to really dissect the science behind fasting and the facts that surround this type of diet plan.

What happens during intermittent fasting?

After a meal is consumed, glucose (sugar) is immediately used as an internal energy source and what is left in the body is stored as fat. The body's fat is then stored in the adipose tissue. During a period of fasting that lasts longer than 8 to 12 hours, you switch from glucose (sugar from the liver) as the main energy source and suddenly use fatty acids and ketones (made from the body's naturally stored fat) as an alternative energy source. These ketones are not only a source of energy but have the role of a signal molecule in the body. As a result, they have an important influence on all cells and organs in our body, especially on the production and activity of proteins and molecules that influence the metabolism.

This internal productivity taking place in your body leads to an increase in the activity of antioxidants in blood cells which in turn has a protective effect against the harmful free radicals in our body. Those antioxidants also ensure repair of DNA, clean up damaged proteins, stimulate the production of mitochondria (which is necessary for energy production) and reduce inflammatory reactions. In addition to serving as an energy source, ketones has a positive effect on the health and aging of our body. They also stimulate the production of a specific substance in the brain (BNDP, a brain-derived neurotrophic factor), which affects the overall health and resilience of our brain.

What health effects does intermittent fasting have?

Many health effects of intermittent fasting have primarily been found from research done with animals, especially mice and rats. Research shows that in healthy animals, there was an obvious improvement in physical ability with the lab animals experiencing better stamina, balance and coordination. Great improvements were also found in the area of cognition, memory and the executive functions (these include planning, organizing and making decisions). In addition to the research, there was seemingly a delay in the aging process. The animals lived longer. There has been a lot of variation on how great this effect is on aging. Some reports show an increase of up to 45% depending on the research given and read. When investigating the effect of intermittent fasting on various cancers, there appears to be the development of fewer tumors, a decrease in the growth of all existing tumors and an increase in the sensitivity of the tumor to chemotherapy and radiation.

There are currently a number of clinical trial studies investigating the effect of fasting in people with cancer. Further, an improvement in physical health has been discovered in animals dealing with multiple sclerosis and rheumatoid arthritis which is probably due to the decrease in inflammatory reactions during fasting. Animals also suffering from neurodegenerative disorders such as Alzheimer's and Parkinson's exhibited positive effects from fasting as shown from a delay in their existing conditions from worsening.

In humans who have lost weight due to intermittent fasting also improved the health of their heart and blood vessels. Such improvements include: lower blood pressure, a resting heart rate, low cholesterol and resistance to triglycerides, glucose and insulin (this also refers to people with pre-stage diabetes and those who already have the disease). These improvements are reported about 2 to 4 weeks after starting intermittent fasting and suddenly disappear when the normal diet returns. The effect of fasting seems to be more than just weight loss. There was a clinical study showing overweight women in which two groups (one with and one without intermittent fasting) received the same number of calories to consume. The weight loss was the same in both groups, but the group engaging in intermittent fasting had an obvious decrease in insulin resistance and a greater reduction in hip size. There are, however, actual studies done which show only weight reduction results without an actual effect on insulin resistance.

What breaks the fast?

All food and drink that contain calories break a fast. Fortunately, in addition to water, a few other options are allowed. Carbonated water is highly suggested for its simplistic bubbles and no sugars or flavors. One common question: can you drink coffee and tea during the fast? Black coffee and tea are allowed! They are both drinks primarily without calories. I would advise you to drink coffee and tea *without* milk and sugar. I personally like to drink 2 to 3 cups of coffee during my fast, the hot beverage makes it more pleasant for me. The caffeine from my coffee is also nice and gives the overall fat-burning a little extra boost.

You can also take supplements during intermittent fasting. Keep in mind that some supplements can irritate the consumer on an empty stomach, causing headaches or stomach problems. Save those supplements for when you eat meals. You can take supplements during your fast, as long as they do not contain calories.

When to not engage in intermittent fasting

Intermittent fasting is not suitable for the following reasons:

- If you are pregnant or breastfeeding
- If you are using medicines that conflict with each other (consult your doctor)
- If you have a history of eating disorders
- If you are experiencing persistent (sleeping) problems during fasting

If you notice that you are not responding well to intermittent fasting, it is better to stop the diet plan immediately. As popular as fasting is, it may not be the ideal diet. Every person is different when it comes to fasting. As a personal experiment, I tried intermittent fasting for 6 weeks and by the 3rd week, I was already used to the diet and made it a regular part of my lifestyle. I will further explain the effects on my body, the results and how I got used to it more in this book.

More FAQs on Intermittent Fasting

Intermittent fasting is not a new concept, but there are certainly questions about this diet plan. Hopefully you can find the answers to some of your questions in these chapters.

How did I get used to intermittent fasting?

I started with the 16/ 8 method where I would only eat for 8 hours a day and it was a little challenging in the beginning. I noticed that if I got hungry at 9:30AM, my hunger disappeared automatically. After about 3 weeks, I was completely adapted to my fasting method and used my job as a good distraction. I always have plenty to do at work. If I start something, I like to finish it and that determined mindset gave me the confidence I needed to continue my diet plan successfully.

Can you lose weight with intermittent fasting?

With intermittent fasting, you can lose weight. Fasting every other day leads to even greater weight loss than casual intermittent fasting due to a low energy intake throughout the week.

Values in the blood

Intermittent fasting may have beneficial effects on some values in the blood. The triglyceride concentration (fat cells in the blood) drops in many case studies and is related to weight loss. Reduction in overall cholesterol and LDL cholesterol has been found in some studies as well. Blood pressure drops if there is sufficient weight loss. Data on the long-term effects of intermittent fasting on health and disease risk are very limited. It is not possible to indicate whether intermittent fasting will cause long-term health risks or health benefits.

Nutritional advice

It is important to get enough nutrients in your body on the days you choose to eat. With intermittent fasting, you don't necessarily need to change your eating habits but certainly choose a responsible diet plan which allows you to lose weight slowly and still get all your nutrients.

Chapter 3

How to Start Intermittent Fasting

Although the concept is simple, it is not easy to start fasting. In our current culture, we are very used to eating three meals a day with snacks which is difficult to change. Most people experience hunger pains, irritability and a decreased ability to concentrate during their periods of fasting. These side effects usually disappear within a month. It is important to consult a nutritionist or dietician so that you do eat enough nutrients during your fast.

In several animal studies and in a number of human clinical trials, intermittent fasting show many health effects. However, more research still needs to be done on this subject. It is not quite clear on the effects of long-term fasting or whether all positive effects found in animals will also apply to humans or if the clinical test results apply to everyone or only to specific groups of people. So, we rely on future studies to show us more about our meals, our food intake and our fasting schedules.

You don't necessarily need anything to start intermittent fasting but I would recommend that you consider the following questions:

- What is your personal goal with intermittent fasting?
- Do you expect to stick to the fasting schedule you created?
- Do you fall into one of the risk groups?

When you start intermittent fasting, make sure you continue your diet plan for at least 2 weeks and preferably up to a month. In the first few days, fasting will take some getting used to and skipping meals is not pleasant. Only after a while will you master this diet and start to reap the health benefits. The most important thing is to maintain a healthy lifestyle whether you eat or fast. Intermittent fasting can sound exciting yet it can be tricky. From my own experience, I recommend the following steps to get started.

Step 1: Take a critical look at your diet and lifestyle

Besides fasting, are there dietary needs you can improve on? Work on these issues immediately. Limit your intake of sugar, carbs and junk food. Stop eating unhealthy snacks after meals. Get enough sleep. The better prepared you are, the greater the chance of success at your fasting diet plan.

Step 2: Create a feasible diet plan

Everyone wants results quickly but ease into this new diet. For example, start with the 12/12 method, where you can eat from 7:00AM to 7:00PM (or whatever times suit you best). With this method, you can still have breakfast and dinner. Or use the 6/1 method in the beginning. In the first few weeks, you only have to stick to the plan for 1 day.

Step 3: Let yourself relax on the weekend

Keep the 12/12 fasting schedule (or whichever fasting method you choose) disciplined until the weekend. On the weekend, let go of the fast and just eat when you want. You deserve that relaxation. This way, even if you are having a difficult time on your fasting diet plan during the week, you always have the weekend to look forward to.

Step 4: Build the intensity at your pace

Are you doing well on the 12/12 method? Just stay at the 12/12 as long as you want. Everyone reacts to this diet at his or her own pace. You might be able to go further on your fast in the coming weeks.

Tips for Intermittent Fasting

I have listed the most effective tips for maintaining intermittent fasting as well as advice to keep the diet a fun experience.

Tip 1: Hunger passes

Are you hungry at 9:00AM and have to wait until 12:00PM to eat? Try to find a distraction. You will notice that after a while, the hunger disappears by itself.

Tip 2: Don't be too hard on yourself

Start your fasting diet plan slowly. Don't be too hard on yourself right away but be careful not to get too relaxed, either. Demand discipline and perseverance from yourself. Do your utmost to keep your diet plan on track and your personal success will taste all the sweeter!

Tip 3: Healthy eating makes it easier

When you are finally allowed to eat, you may be wanting to reach for the unhealthy foods. Do not do this! You will make your fasting diet more difficult to maintain. Nutrient-rich, high-fat (good fats) and low-carbohydrate foods make intermittent fasting much easier to continue.

Tip 4: Use caution when exercising

Sports and intermittent fasting go well together. If you are just starting to fast your meals, be very careful with physical exercise. Your body needs time to adapt to this new diet. I do not recommend a high intensity workout during fasting. A light workout or walk is a good alternative. If you feel dizzy, have a headache or other complaints, then don't exercise. Don't be too hard on yourself when first starting out. If you make it unnecessarily strenuous on yourself, you may not be able to maintain your fasting regime.

Tip 5: Drink enough

Drink enough water during your fast. You can also drink beverages without calories (coffee or tea), just make sure you drink 1.5 to 2 liters of water a day!

Tip 6: Stay disciplined to fasting

When you yield to just one cookie, then your body starts all kinds of processes and reacts to the food consumption all over again. Resist temptation and stick to a glass of water when you feel the need to eat.

Tip 7: Give yourself enough time to get used to it

I disciplined myself and maintained my fasting diet for 6 weeks. After those 6 weeks, I decided whether I wanted to continue or not. I recommend that you try your diet for at *least* 3 weeks. You don't want to drop out just before you experience the full health benefits of fasting.

Tip 8: Coffee takes away the feeling of hunger

If you like coffee, you're in luck! Coffee beverages take away the feeling of hunger. Tea can also have this effect and it is a nice change from just drinking water.

Tip 9: Distraction takes away the feeling of hunger

The easiest days to fast are the days you are working. During the week, I have enough distractions at the office to help take my mind off my hunger pains. Before I know it, it is lunch time and I can eat again.

Tip 10: Fasting is not for everyone

No matter how beneficial fasting can be, it is not for everyone. Every person is different. If fasting doesn't work for you, just remember that there are countless ways to live a healthy life!

How to Practice Intermittent Fasting?

Before starting any new eating regime, it is important to speak to your doctor and make sure it is safe for your lifestyle and dietary needs. "Fasting can affect blood sugar levels and leave certain populations more at risk. If you are pregnant, have any health conditions, especially diabetes, heart conditions or are prone to low blood sugar, this diet is risky," says a medical expert. She also recommends that people who take medicines that need to be taken with a meal consult a physician before attempting intermittent fasting. "Anyone with disordered eating should avoid any strict diet, intermittent fasting included," adds a medical expert. Once you are given the go-ahead by your healthcare provider, here's how to get started:

- ***Pick the fasting method that works best for you.*** Review your current lifestyle and eating habits to decide which strategy best fits your life. Do you have some jam-packed workdays where you hardly have time to eat? You may want to try the modified fasting method, where you eat limited calories two days a week. If you're never in the mood for breakfast, you might want to try the time-limited approach, eating only in the afternoon and early evening. Begin with a fasting diet plan you think will work best for you and switch to another method if you need to.

- ***Realize that your obsessive food thoughts will pass!*** Many newbies to this eating style admit that the first days can be rough and fantasizing about food is common about a week into intermittent fasting. Your hunger pains should drop, your energy levels should be consistent and you'll find out quickly if this fasting diet plan is right for you.

- ***Slowly exercise on fasting days.*** Most people who practice intermittent fasting work out regularly. A medical expert comments on this, "You might feel hungry after a workout, so it might not be enjoyable to do it on a full fasting day. Walking, yoga, and stretching on fasting days could be better to avoid any negative side effects." If you are engaging in a limited fasting, it might be best to save your exercise session for right before breaking your fast.

- ***Don't forget to drink up!*** It's important to stay hydrated while fasting; keep your water bottle handy. During your fasting times, you can also enjoy tea or black coffee. Keep in mind that caffeine can have greater effects on an empty stomach, so you might be more prone to shaking or anxiety if you consume too much. Listen to your body and how it feels with this new routine.

Chapter 4

Intermittent Fasting Methods

There are many ways in which you can partake in intermittent fasting. You can occasionally schedule a 24 hour fast from food during which you only drink water or herbal tea. Or you can eat 1 meal a day and drink for the rest, eating usually a lunch or evening meal. Another way to experience intermittent fasting is to only eat within a certain time period of the day, for example, between 8:00AM and 8:00PM. This method means there is 12 hours of eating and 12 hours of fasting. This can be extended to 10 hours of eating and 14 hours of fasting or 8 hours of eating and 16 hours of fasting. A combination of the above methods is also possible.

Intermittent fasting schedules

Intermittent fasting means you eat a certain part of the day or week and refrain from food for the rest of the time. Here are all the fasting schedules to consider:

- The 13/11 schedule: 13 hours of fasting and 11 hours of eating (every day)
- The 14/10 schedule: fast for 14 hours and eat for 10 hours (every day)

- The 16/8 schedule: 16 hours of fasting and 8 hours of eating (every day)
- The 20/4 schedule: 20 hours of fasting and 4 hours of eating (every day)
- OMAD schedule: fasting one meal a day (every day)
- Fasting for 24-36 hours: fasting all day once or twice a week
- The 5/2 schedule: 5 days of eating and 2 days of fasting (every week)

The 13/11 schedule

The 13/11 schedule is the most popular and easily accessible form of fasting. This method involves fasting from food for 13 hours of the day and then eating for the remaining 11 hours. This diet plan is very easy to maintain. You will feel more energetic and better over time.

The 14/10 schedule

This fasting method is just a step up from the 13/11 schedule. It is the right diet plan for you if you want to take things to the next level. Instead of eating breakfast at 8:00AM, you don't eat until 9:00AM or 10:00AM and that extra effort comes with additional benefits. The 14 hours of rest you give your body will give you plenty of extra energy.

The 16/8 schedule

The 16/8 fasting method is the most widely used intermittent fasting method in the world. This diet plan is used by people who want to lose weight and also by athletes and bodybuilders to achieve optimal results. The 16/8 method means that you fast from food for 16 hours in one day and have an eating period of 8 hours. One common way of achieving this diet is to skip breakfast altogether. One example of this method is to start eating at noon and take your last meal at 8:00PM. This schedule has a big impact on your daily life as you would eat your first meal at 12:00PM and have enough time for dinner in the evening. You can expect truly spectacular results such as more energy and diminished health issues. The best results are achieved best if you eat 2 meals in those designated 8 hours.

The 20/4 schedule

The 20/4 fasting diet is a pretty intense method and only a few people can maintain this diet plan for a long amount of time. In the 20/4 schedule, you only have a time frame of 4 hours to eat, usually from 3:00PM to 7:00PM. You can maintain this method several days a week to give your body extra rest, but following this schedule every day is too intense for most people.

OMAD schedule

The term OMAD stands for eating One Meal A Day. You could also call this method the 23/1 schedule, fasting 23 hours from food and eating 1 hour. This diet plan is most effective when you make that one meal your evening meal. This schedule is hard to maintain every day because you consume too few nutrients to continue on a daily basis. Eating only one meal every day is very healthy and also helps you to lose weight.

Fasting for 36 hours

A fast of 36 hours is not only good for your overall health, but it is also very good training for your discipline and will power. With this diet plan, you eat dinner on day 1 around 7:00PM, then you don't eat on day 2 and only on day 3, you eat breakfast at 7:00AM. This means refraining from food for 36 hours. You will notice that on day 2 in the afternoon, you will experience hunger pains. Hunger often goes away by itself. So if you feel hungry, you don't necessarily have to eat!

The 5/2 schedule

With the 5/2 schedule, you eat 5 days a week and then fast 2 days a week. With this method, you experience more peace, feel even better and are not guided by hunger. During a 24 hour fast, your body breaks down some muscles, which can be counterproductive for those people who are trying to build up more muscle mass. There is also a variant of this diet plan where instead of fasting from food for 2 days, you allow yourself to eat one small meal (about 500 to 600 calories per day) on those designated days.

24 hour fasting schedule

This fasting method is very simple to follow. You don't eat anything for 24 hours, 1 to 2 times a week. This diet plan usually means fasting from dinner to dinner. You can also fast from breakfast to breakfast or from lunch to lunch. This schedule is not for beginners and I do not recommend this method if you have never done intermittent fasting before. The last few hours of a 24 hour fast are not always easy. A 12/12 or 16/8 fasting method is a better step for beginners. Do you want to use the 24 hour fasting method to lose weight? I would suggest eating normal in preparation for the fast day and do not fill up completely on food. Eat healthy and no more than you would normally eat.

Flexible fasting method

This is not an official method, but just a name I made up. Are you unable to consistently maintain a fasting diet plan? Then you can fast in a more flexible way. Skip a breakfast every now and then. Do not eat anything after dinner and eat breakfast a little later the following day. Choose to eat only 2 small meals in a day. In this way, you will not experience all the health benefits and you will not get used to fasting, but you will take away small bits of profit.

Be easy on yourself

If you're comfortable with your chosen fasting plan, maintain your method several days a week. If you have fluctuating blood sugar levels and find it difficult to continue without breakfast, eat an early evening meal that ends at 6:00PM. If you don't eat anything until 8:00AM the next day, you would have fasted for 14 hours which is an excellent start!

Build things up slowly

If you have stable blood sugar, you can choose to eat early in the evening and delay eating your breakfast. If you finish your dinner at 7:00PM and start breakfast at 11:00AM, you would have fasted 16 hours. You can do this as often as you like. This is my favorite fasting method, I do this four to five times a week. Sometimes I skip breakfast and have lunch around noon.

If your normal fasting period is for only 8 hours, expand this to 12 hours. From there you can stretch it a little further. Do not fast from food 7 days a week! Keep surprising your body again and again and eat at varying times. The greatest benefits of intermittent fasting will only be obtained if you eat as healthy as possible and if you eat less than usual. Stay disciplined before the fasting period begins, especially if you want to lose weight.

Expectations with intermittent fasting

Intermittent fasting will give you several positive health benefits. I want to break down the three most prominent effects.

Fat burning and muscle maintenance. In two months, I lost about 3 to 4 kilos, which was almost completely fat. I also managed to maintain my muscle mass during fasting. I lost weight but my muscle mass and strength remained at the same level.

More energy and better stamina. It sounds almost contradictory, but by not eating breakfast, I feel even more energy, both in my body and in my mind. My energy levels are now much more stable. In addition, my stamina when running has improved even after two weeks of intermittent fasting.

Less dependent on food. Before my intermittent fasting diet plan, I was quite dependent on my meals. I could hardly function without breakfast or dinner. Now, after a few weeks of intermittent fasting, if I have dinner much later or skip lunch, that's no problem. Once a month, I go on a 24 hour fast. I have definitely become much less dependent on food consumption.

When is intermittent fasting not a good idea?

In theory, anyone can be on an intermittent fasting diet plan. Our bodies can naturally cope with long periods without food. However, there are groups of people that should not be fasting.

- Women who are pregnant or breastfeeding

- People with a current or past history of eating disorders
- People who experience a lot of stress
- Older people who naturally consume fewer calories

I also advise people who take heavy medications to contact their doctor before they start with intermittent fasting.

Not for everyone: your body is always right

It remains important to use your common sense when fasting. It may not be a good idea to fast if you are recovering from surgery, have an illness, are pregnant or already low in weight. If you are addicted to sugar or your blood glucose levels fluctuate considerably, then your body will benefit more from eating regularly. Build up intermittent fasting very slowly or omit it completely. Work on stabilizing your blood sugar and training your body to use fat molecules as a source of energy.

Chapter 5

The Benefits of Intermittent Fasting

Now that you know the different methods of intermittent fasting, it's time to take a look at the benefits it can bring. Scientific research has been conducted on intermittent fasting for decades. These studies show that there are many health benefits for not eating during a certain period (14 hours or more). The good news is that intermittent fasting gives you more energy and that's why I'm such an advocate.

Intermittent fasting increases insulin sensitivity

The less insulin you need to get 1 unit of glucose from your blood, the higher your insulin sensitivity. People who are insulin resistant have low insulin sensitivity. This means that they need a lot of insulin to filter 1 unit of glucose from their blood. Insulin resistance creates a lot of health problems. The best known is type 2 diabetes. However, insulin resistance often plays an important role in obesity, as well. By maintaining a intermittent fasting diet plan, you increase your insulin sensitivity (2 GB), which is very healthy. A vital side note here is that the type of food you do eat should be low in carbohydrates, natural and unprocessed. If you eat a lot of sugars, the blood sugar can worsen by eating less often.

Intermittent fasting increases fat burning

Intermittent fasting helps you lose weight, especially if you consume healthy food during those eating times. If you eat low-carb, natural and unprocessed food, you will consume fewer calories and burn stored body fat. Intermittent fasting also improves certain hormone functions. You will experience lower insulin levels, higher growth hormone levels and an increase in norepinephrine (noradrenaline). All of this leads to breaking down more body fat for energy and makes you lose weight faster. A clinical study in 2014 concluded that with intermittent fasting, you could burn between 3-8% body fat in just 3 weeks.

Most people who try intermittent fasting want to lose weight. When you have a small eating time period in one day, you have less time to eat fewer meals and less meals mean fewer calories. You should not eat extra during those pre-ordained meal times. Your hormones will be in the right position for fat burning.

Intermittent fasting ensures good cholesterol

Fasting can have a positive effect on cholesterol and triglyceride levels. Several studies have shown that intermittent fasting improves the relationship between LDL (bad cholesterol) and HDL (good cholesterol). When you follow a well-balanced diet while fasting, the effects on your cholesterol are even better.

Intermittent fasting improves heart and blood vessels

Many studies, primarily with animals, reveal that intermittent fasting positively influence a large number of indicators for cardiovascular problems with a healthier cholesterol level with an anti-inflammatory effect. This diet plan reduces oxidative stress in the body. Intermittent fasting helps inhibit inflammation and enables you to have a healthier cardiovascular system.

A longer life

Intermittent fasting is the ultimate dream of all anti-aging gurus because intermittent fasting seems to extend the lifespan. Studies show that with intermittent fasting, you can extend life and calorie restriction. In case studies, some lab rats lived up to 80% longer meaning the chance is higher in the life expectancy in humans especially considering the other benefits that intermittent fasting creates. Our body is constantly busy with internal processes which releases free radicals, substances that are harmful to us. The first step towards aging and various chronic diseases is an excess of free radicals and oxidative stress. Intermittent fasting strengthens our body's resistance to oxidative stress. According to research, intermittent fasting helps fight inflammation which is considered another important factor to many diseases.

Intermittent fasting is good for the brain

You already read that fasting is good for your metabolism and hormone balance. This diet plan also reduces oxidative stress and inflammation which is not only good for the body but also for your brain. Research on rats shows that intermittent fasting enhances the growth of new nerve cells. People with a shortage of the BDNF level, a brain-derived neurotrophic factor, often have to deal with depression or mental issues.

Pitfalls with intermittent fasting

There are many health benefits of intermittent fasting, but it's not for everyone! Here are some possible disadvantages to intermittent fasting.

Not suitable for all athletes

During fasting, you do not eat during long periods of the day and your body cannot always produce an optimal amount of energy. Athletes may experience less performance and productivity in their workouts. Some athletes however report that intermittent fasting actually improves their performance.

Caution in people using medication

When you use medication, it is always wise to consult your doctor first before engaging in a fasting diet plan. Some medications need an active metabolism or full stomach to work properly.

Eating too much and consuming the wrong foods

Some people view intermittent fasting as permission to consume unhealthy food during those periods when they can eat. This will be counterproductive to achieve those personal fasting goals. Some people cannot resist the feeling of hunger during a fast and eat a lot of unhealthy food in a binge.

Dropout percentage is high

If you do engage in one of the more intense forms of intermittent fasting, the chances are that you will eventually give up on day 3 or 4 because of the difficultly of the diet. If you get through days 3, 4, and 5, it will be much easier to continue your fast! I advise people to start with a 13/11 fasting schedule and then slowly build up the number of hours of refraining from food. This way it's easier and you still enjoy many of the health benefits.

Investigations are still in progress

The positive results of intermittent fasting are very promising. However, many of the clinical studies have been done on animals, not humans. I recommend you try intermittent fasting for yourself for at least 2 weeks and discover the personal improvements over your mind, body and spirit.

Conclusion

Having touched on all the intermittent fasting methods along with the health benefits and potential risks associated with fasting, you are now equipped with the right tools to help you on your fasting adventure. I can't promise you it will be easy, but with the right attitude and determination, you are going to see substantial results.

The first few days and weeks on your fasting diet plan might be a little difficult as your body adjusts to your new regime, but don't worry. You will be able to figure out the perfect fasting schedule that works best for you. Be sure to consult your doctor if you'd like to try the fasting diet plan and prepare for amazing health benefits!

www.ingramcontent.com/pod-product-compliance
Ingram Content Group UK Ltd.
Pitfield, Milton Keynes, MK11 3LW, UK
UKHW020136250726
13967UKWH00002B/696